Healing Words & Heartfelt Care

A Guided Journal for Healthcare Professionals

By Dr. Tishon Creswell

Healing Words & Heartfelt Care

Copyright © 2023 by Tishon Creswell.

No part of this book may be used or reproduced in any manner whatsoever without the prior written permission of the author.

To request permissions, contact the publisher at iamtishon@gmail.com.

Dedication

This journal is dedicated to the healthcare professionals who tirelessly serve as the pillars of compassion and healing. May these unseen heroes find inspiration and resilience within these words, reflecting their immeasurable impact.

Introduction

Introducing a transformative self-care journal designed exclusively for healthcare professionals. Navigate the challenges of your noble profession with introspective journaling, mindful reflection, and fortified resilience. Elevate your well-being, rekindle your passion, and empower your journey in healthcare through the pages of this essential companion.

Remember, this journal is your companion on a path of self-discovery and renewal. By completing it at your own pace, you're honoring your individual needs and creating space for transformative growth on your terms. Grab your colored pencils to engage in self-care coloring activities sprinkled throughout.

-Dr. Tishon Creswell

What was the defining moment or experience that led you to choose a healthcare career?

Describe the ways you've grown since your first day in healthcare.

Write about a mentor who guided and shaped you on your journey.

Write about the qualities that make you a unique and valued healthcare professional.

How has your initial aspiration to become a healthcare professional evolved?

Describe a skill you've developed on your healthcare journey. How has it evolved?

What values and principles do you hold dear as a healthcare professional? How do these values guide your decisions and actions?

What role does self-care play in your life as a healthcare professional?

How do you prioritize your own well-being amidst the demands of your career?

Describe the role of self-care in maintaining your professional standards.

Discuss the small moments of joy you find amidst the chaos of healthcare.

REMINDER

Taking care of yourself is productive

TIME FOR A STRETCH BREAK

1. While sitting or standing, relax your shoulders.
2. Reach your right arm across your chest at shoulder height.
3. Use your left arm to gently pull it closer against your chest and hold for about one minute.
4. Release, and switch arms.
5. Repeat as needed.

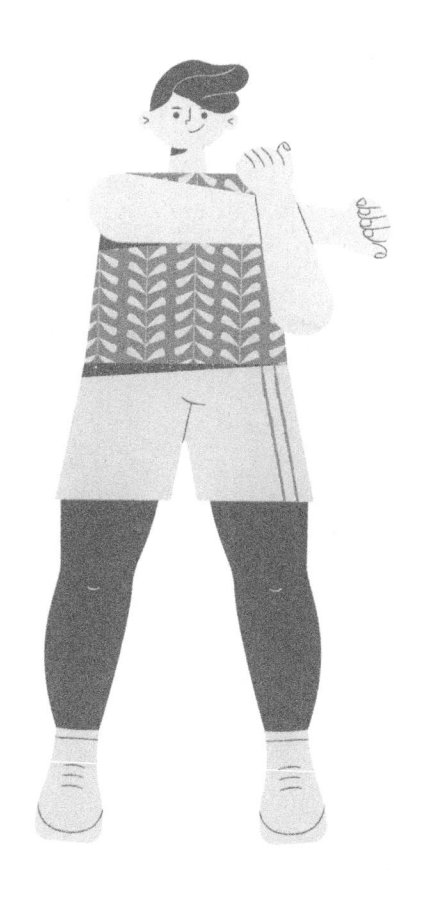

"Nurses dispense comfort, compassion, and caring without even a prescription."

-Val Saintsbury

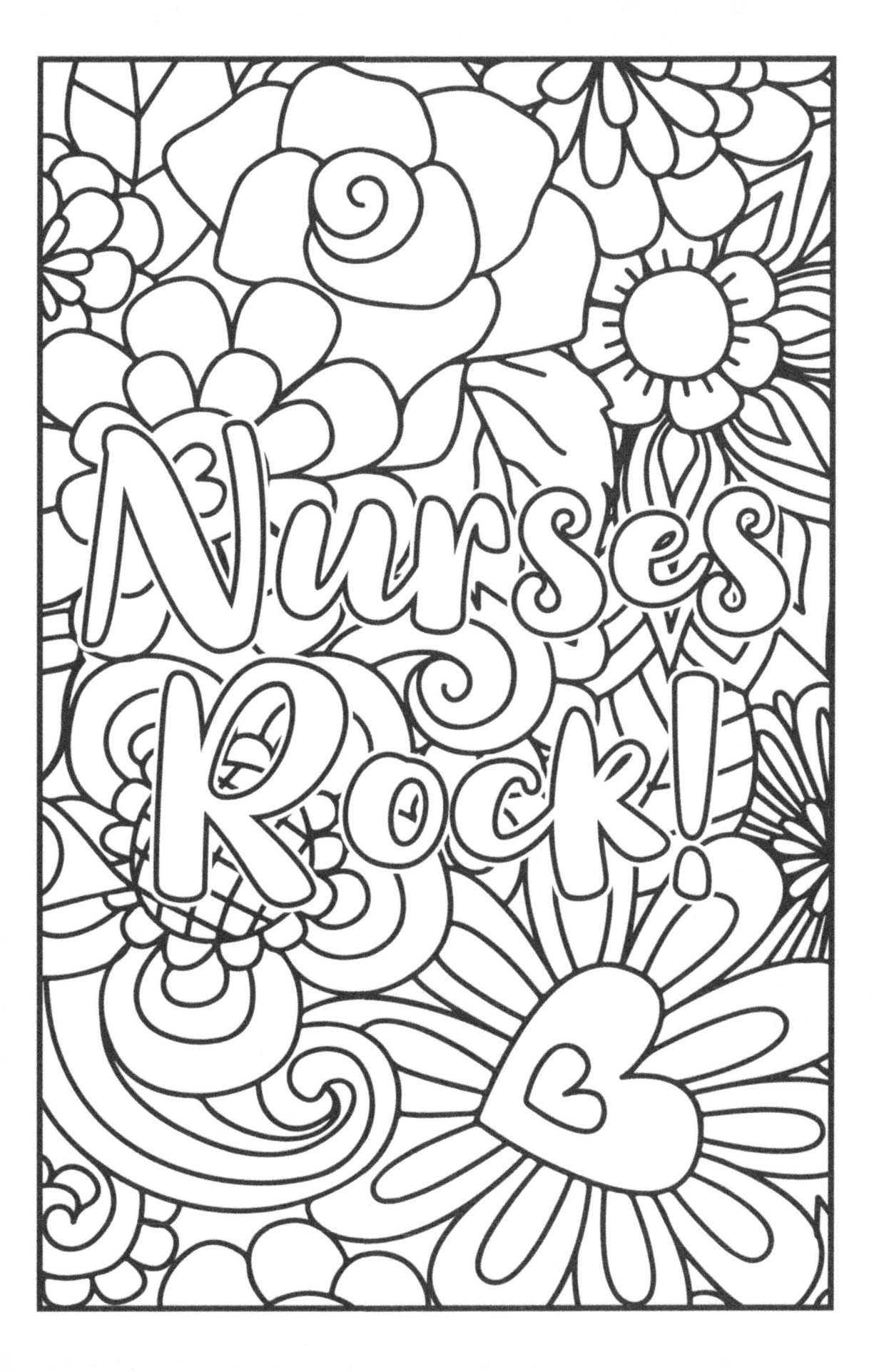

How can you prioritize self-care to prevent burnout?

Describe the impact of long working hours on your mental and physical well-being.

Discuss the importance of work-life balance in your demanding field.

Reflect on the impact of your profession on your sleep patterns. What changes can you make to prioritize rest and rejuvenation?

Describe the importance of setting boundaries with co-workers to maintain a healthy work-life balance.

Describe a moment when you felt overwhelmed by the demands of your job.

What strategies can you implement to manage your workload more effectively?

Describe an instance when you recognized the early signs of burnout in yourself.

What steps did you take to regain balance?

How has the stress at work affected your home life?

Describe a time when you felt isolated or alone in your struggle with stress or anxiety.

self-care

/ˌselfˈker/ noun

the practice of taking action to preserve or improve one's own health.

SELF-CARE BINGO

Complete one activity daily, weekly, or monthly

Take a walk during lunch	Dance to your favorite song	Make a new recipe	Listen to a podcast	Treat yourself to a massage
Spend 30 min on a hobby	Read a book	Take a power nap	Sit on porch or under a tree	Eat lunch with a friend
Take a day off social media	Say "NO"	Free Space	Soak in bathtub	Buy yourself something nice
Take the stairs at work	Declutter work bag	Treat yourself to a pedicure	Pack a healthy lunch	Meditation
Go to the salon or barber	Go see a movie	Flirt with your self in the mirror	Color or put together a puzzle	Organize closet or drawer

Words of Affirmation "You are....."

```
A X S L I V A G B P F G K H D M D G A G G
T F S J G G G L Q E H R T I Q W F H A C V N
A H X K D I N B U U A G Y M K K X U T F Y O
K I N D F Y X I E F L U U N Q V H M B H G R
O P L Y W C N O R M E J T O G D E V A R B T
G J Y L O V I N G A O T D I N H Y L L F Q S
J T S T C G H D X H C S A E F E N B V D G O
L T A U G L Y Y D L M B E R R U P O Y K D P
W L R Y C U G M T W Y J B W G I L T M G W Q
E X V F I C D N M P A T E J A X P Y V P O C
E W M K N Y E M H V E T N V A H E S P A R S
K T N O H D T S E L R R Q E I U D R N F T A
B Y F M I O F D S P R W S E I T J A L I H K
S T R F Q W P E C F F N V F U L A F O W L M
X F N P W M R E A U U J R S E L I E M H Y D
R O Y H R Q H L F R Y L W E G U G S R T E L
C X L R D O V E S U L V I X P F K J E C L Q
T T D J T L U D V S L E F J W R U N E R G B
L O L R O X I D G Y P L S Q H E K S T M U P
E S A M U D V M L G T W Y S L W P I D V D Y
R M P S S P T A N M O Y F K O O T I A S O P
S A P T F J W E J G J S V R P P R K B F V A
```

POWERFUL	KIND	LOVING	SMART
RESILIENT	PROUD	BEAUTIFUL	FEARLESS
GRATEFUL	BRAVE	CONFIDENT	AWESOME
STRONG	CARING	WORTHLY	SUCCESSFUL
INSPIRED	CREATIVE	HOPEFUL	ENOUGH

Have a heart!

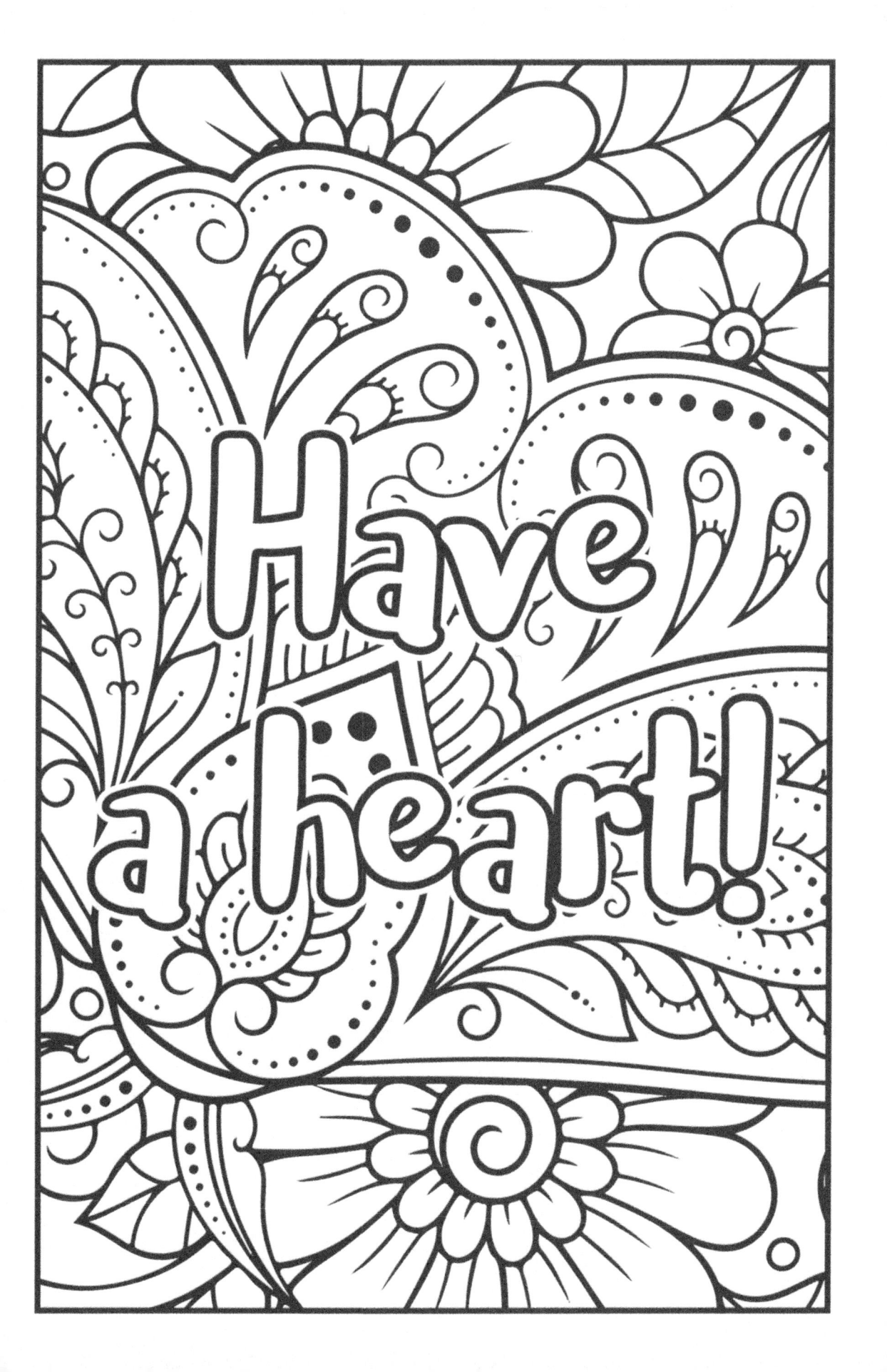

How can you reach out for support and create a network of understanding peers?

Discuss the role of exercise and physical activity in managing stress and anxiety.

How can you incorporate movement into your daily routine, even during busy shifts?

Discuss the concept of seeking professional help when dealing with prolonged stress, anxiety, or depression.

_____
_____
_____
_____
_____
_____
_____
_____
_____
_____
_____
_____
_____
_____
_____
_____
_____
_____
_____
_____
_____
_____

What barriers might prevent you from seeking assistance, and how can you overcome them?

_____
_____
_____
_____
_____
_____
_____
_____
_____
_____
_____
_____
_____
_____
_____
_____
_____
_____
_____
_____

Describe a time when you found solace in creative expression or a hobby outside of work.

How can you carve out more time for these activities to nurture your mental health?

Describe the power of gratitude in counteracting stress and depression.

_____
_____
_____
_____
_____
_____
_____
_____
_____
_____
_____
_____
_____
_____
_____
_____
_____
_____
_____
_____

How can you cultivate a practice of acknowledging positive moments in your day?

Describe a moment when you felt the weight of responsibility as a healthcare provider.

How did you rise to the occasion, and how did it shape your sense of accountability?

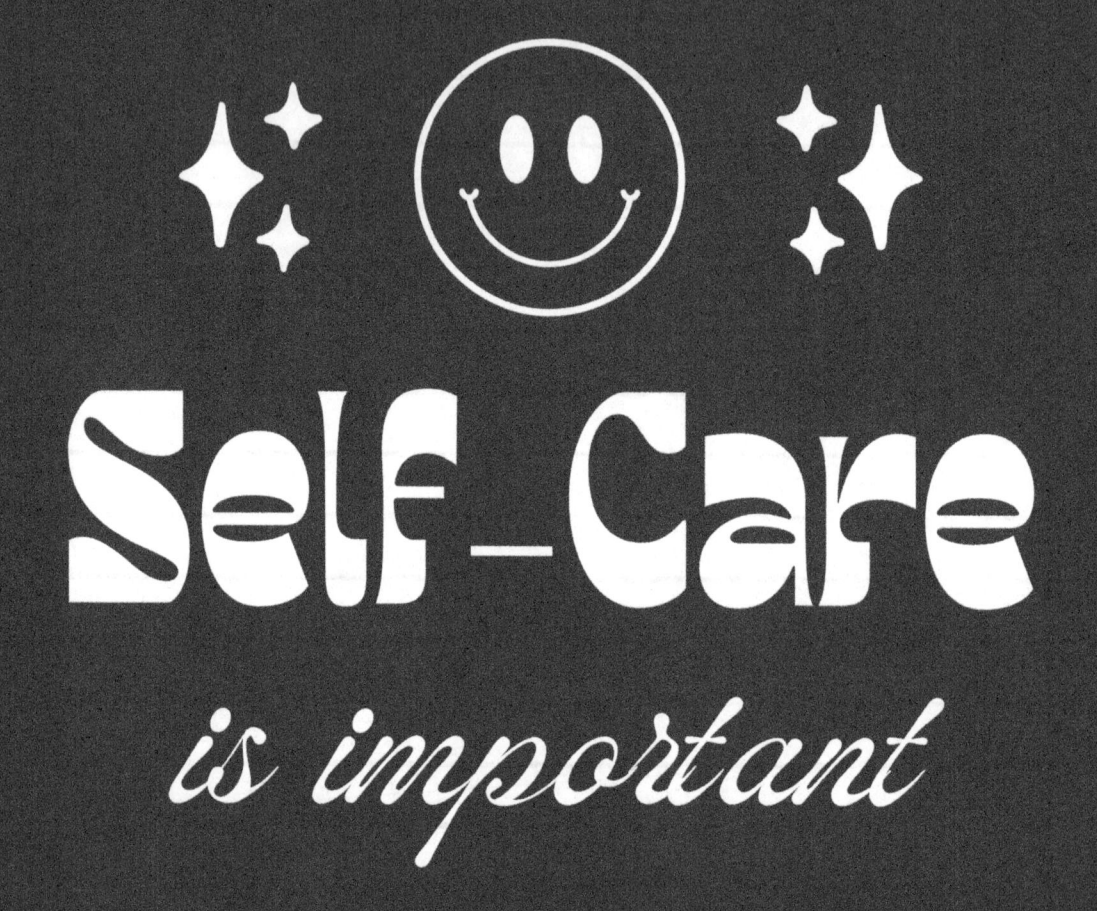

Self-Care

is important

TIME FOR A STRETCH BREAK

1. Feet shoulder width apart, arms at sides.
2. With one hand, reach up overhead and slowly lean towards opposite side. Keep both feet flat on the ground.
3. Hold for 15-30 seconds.
4. Return to starting position and repeat 3-5 times on each side.

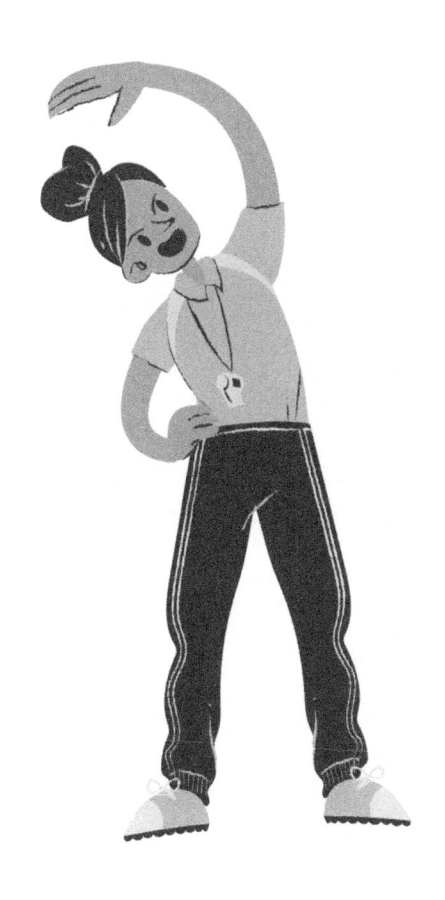

"Every patient carries her or his own doctor inside."

-Albert Schweitzer

Doctors Save Lives!

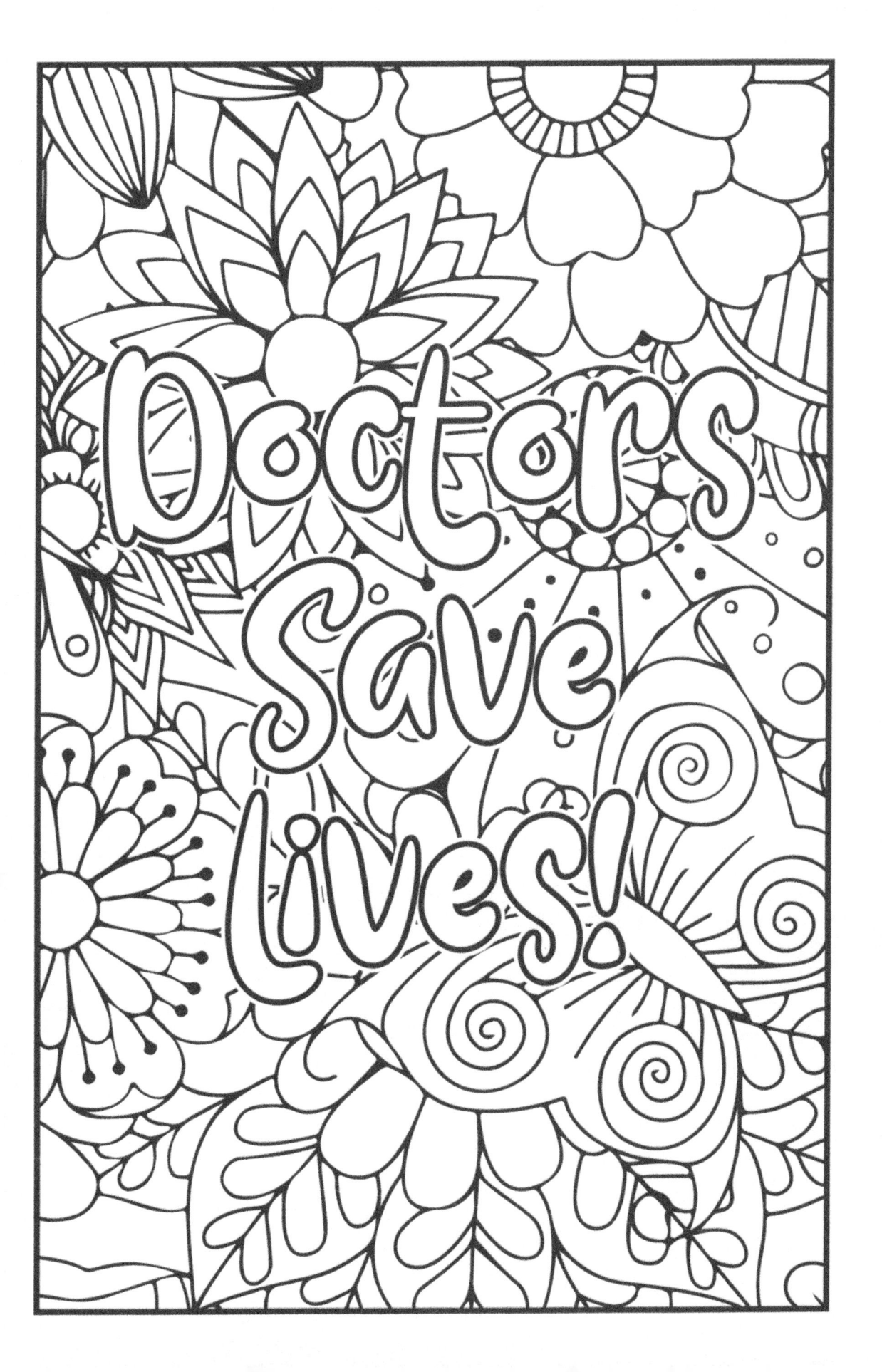

Describe a patient interaction that touched your heart. How did it impact you?

Describe a coworker who inspires you and the qualities you admire in them.

Describe a situation that made you question your resilience. How did you bounce back?

_____
_____
_____
_____
_____
_____
_____
_____
_____
_____
_____
_____
_____
_____
_____
_____
_____
_____
_____
_____
_____

Write a gratitude list, focusing on the elements of your job that bring you fulfillment.

Reflect on a time when you advocated for a patient's needs. How did it make you feel?

Describe a self-care ritual you cherish during your breaks.

_____
_____
_____
_____
_____
_____
_____
_____
_____
_____
_____
_____
_____
_____
_____
_____
_____
_____

Reflect on the challenges of teamwork in healthcare. How do you contribute to a harmonious environment?

___

Reflect on a patient outcome that reaffirmed your dedication to healthcare.

Describe a situation where you had to convey difficult news to a patient's family.

Write about a time when you had to balance empathy with maintaining professional boundaries.

Explore a fear or insecurity related to your profession. How can you work to overcome it?

_____
_____
_____
_____
_____
_____
_____
_____
_____
_____
_____
_____
_____
_____
_____
_____
_____
_____
_____
_____

Self-care
IS EMPOWERMENT

TIME FOR A STRETCH BREAK

1. Holding on for balance with your left hand (optional), grab your right foot or ankle with your right hand.
2. Feel the stretch in the front of your thigh. Hold for 15-30 seconds. Repeat this stretch 3-5 times.
3. Repeat stretch on oppositeleg.

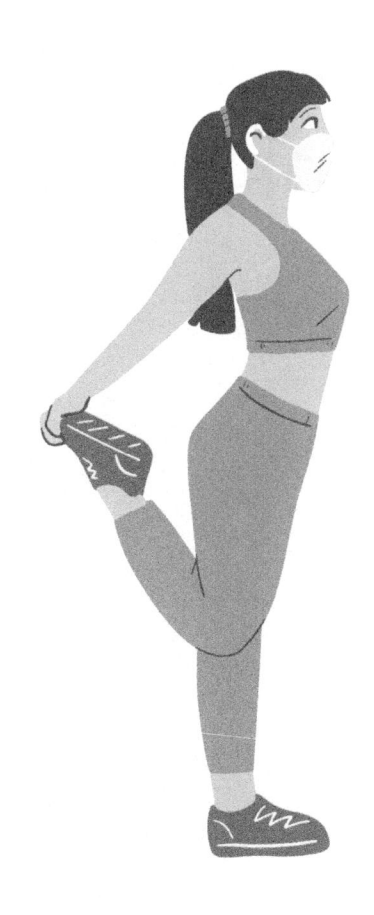

"Social workers advocate for those who have lost their voice, empowering them to reclaim it."

-Unknown

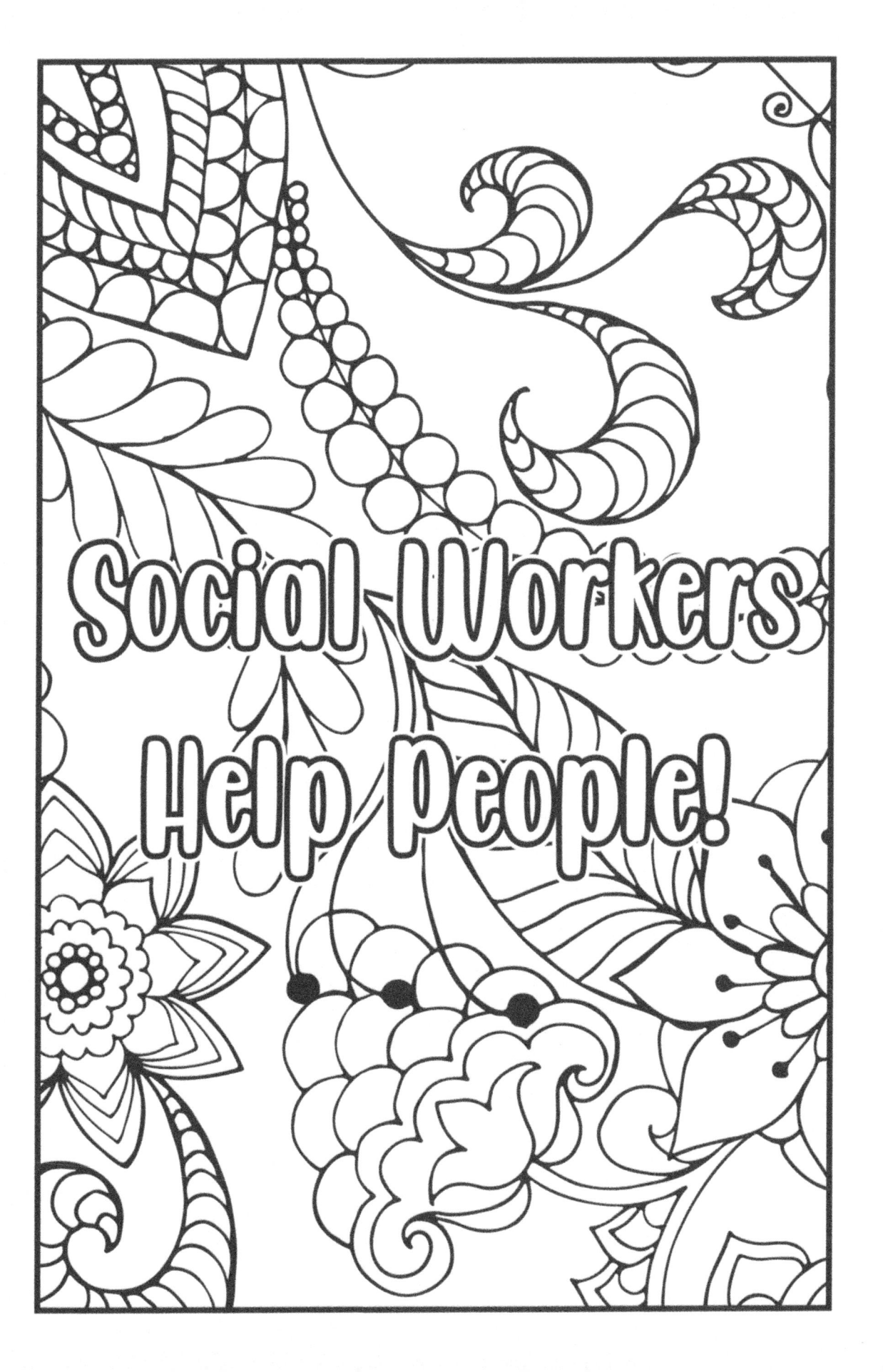

Social Workers Help People!

Describe an instance where you stood up against discrimination or bias in your healthcare setting. How did it impact the situation?

Explore a situation where you felt unfairly treated due to your gender, ethnicity, or other personal characteristics.

How did you find strength in adversity?

Write about a strategy you've used to navigate interactions with difficult co-workers. How can you promote constructive communication?

Describe a time when you felt unsupported by colleagues. How did you cope, and what resources can you tap into for assistance?

Describe an experience when you witnessed someone else being bullied or mistreated at work.

How did you respond, and what could you do differently in the future?

Describe a situation where you had to address a co-worker's inappropriate behavior.

How can you promote a culture of respect and accountability?

Write about a time when you collaborated with co-workers to improve the work environment and foster a sense of unity.

Describe a moment when you collaborated effectively with colleagues to improve patient care.

Take A Break!

SELF-CARE BINGO

Complete one activity daily, weekly, or monthly

Take a walk during lunch	Dance to your favorite song	Make a new recipe	Listen to a podcast	Treat yourself to a massage
Spend 30 min on a hobby	Read a book	Take a power nap	Sit on porch or under a tree	Eat lunch with a friend
Take a day off social media	Say "NO"	Free Space	Soak in bathtub	Buy yourself something nice
Take the stairs at work	Declutter work bag	Treat yourself to a pedicure	Pack a healthy lunch	Meditation
Go to the salon or barber	Go see a movie	Flirt with your self in the mirror	Color or put together a puzzle	Organize closet or drawer

Social Workers, Speech Therapy, Physical Therapy

```
T H D X E C N A L A B F B B I Y L W T O U D
L C S Y I E X K V I P C R D T S J W P G V C
N L G F O R K N B I I H Y I R A S H P G O R
A B N L Y Q S H L U U X N C N D L E G F L I
E H A Y L O F I U G A U A A I Y L G N R T S
C A I N L W P C X H M Q I H X H I X O M Y I
I F E L J T R B S M C L D A Q L K V I G K S
J U M L N W E Y O F N Y S G O X S J T N T S
H R G W V H T C H T Q W O H J L R T A I O T
T M Y C A C O V D A H N H E A T O L C H E R
S E F H N V U G C J N K C B L A T O I C M E
X A D D I C T I O N H F R H C N O N N T P N
I C O G N I T I V E R K M I M K M D U E A G
H V D M I K Y F U I O P S S E B E U M R T T
B I O M E C H A N I C S B H K J N N M T H H
I Y O E P U R E E K Q A A M Q G I X O S Y E
V M L E T L H O O V A I S Q E O F R C F E N
B J G D U D F O X C Q R X E S B B A G N D I
C L M G N I W O L L A W S Q F H U M D Y A N
G R E C O V E R Y G D A H X R W B D C L F G
I W R E A C H E R W N Y S T Q U V T Y U V G
U L S T X H Q F V Y C D I A K C O S W X T Y
```

EMPATHY	ADVOCACY	CRISIS	COMMUNITY
ADDICTION	ICE	BIOMECHANICS	RECOVERY
STRETCHING	BALANCE	STRENGTHENING	HEAT
COGNITIVE	SWALLOWING	PUREE	COMMUNICATION
AIRWAY	FINE MOTOR SKILLS	SOCK AID	REACHER

PT will move you!

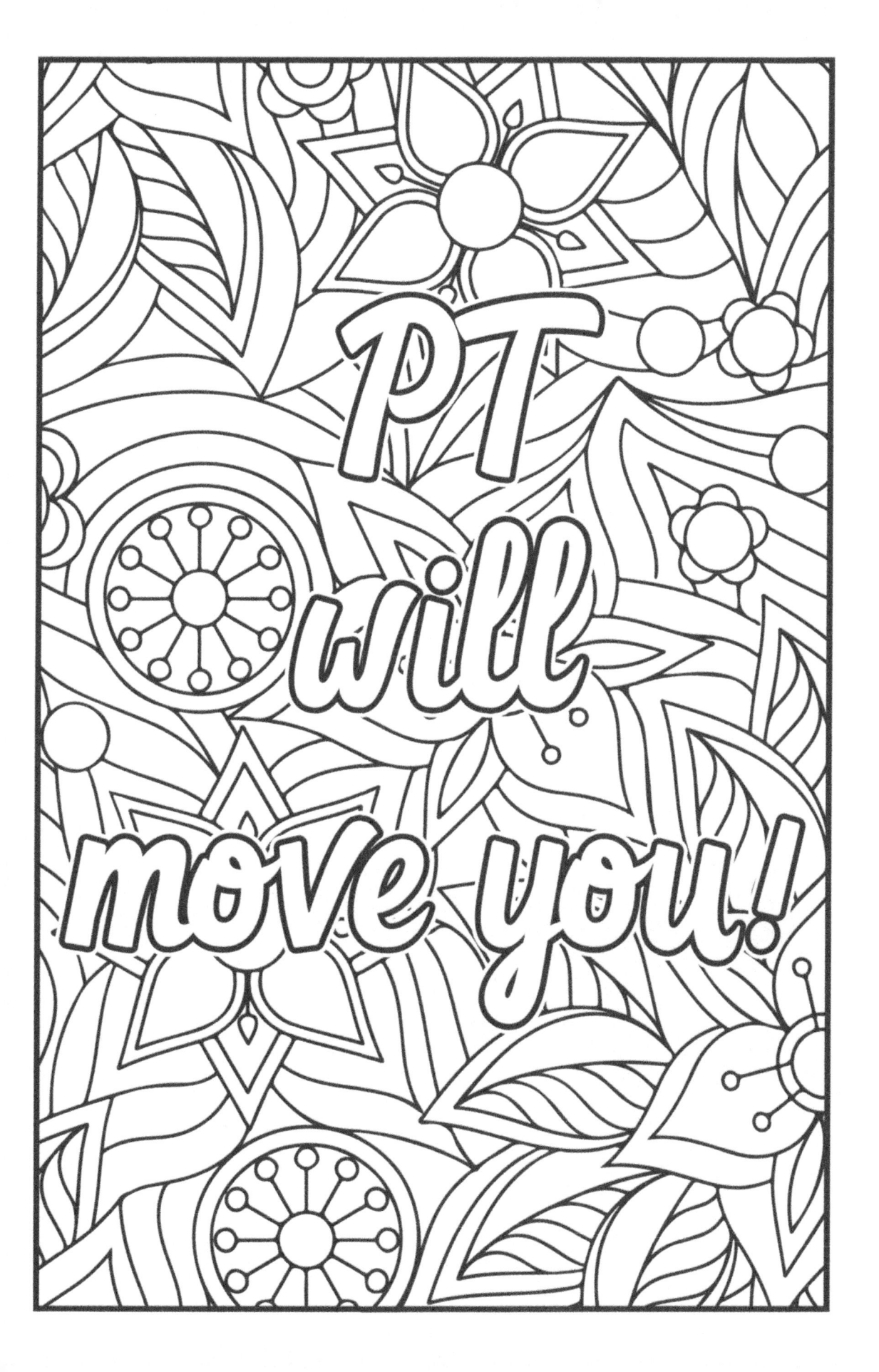

When advocating for your patient's needs within a multidisciplinary team, write about the balance between assertiveness and collaboration.

How can you effectively convey your concerns while maintaining a harmonious environment?

Explore the concept of humility in healthcare interactions. How can you balance advocating for your opinions while remaining open to the insights of others?

Describe the impotantance of the interdisciplinary team's communication in optimizing patient outcomes.

How can you proactively foster open lines of communication with colleagues from diverse backgrounds?

Reflect on a recent collaborative success with a colleague from a different healthcare discipline.

How did effective teamwork enhance patient care, and what lessons can you carry forward?

Describe a challenging encounter with a fellow healthcare professional that tested your communication skills and patience.

How can you apply conflict resolution techniques to navigate such situations in the future?

Describe the connection between your professional identity and your mental well-being.

How can you maintain a strong sense of self while navigating the challenges of your role?

SELF
CARE

Short Self-Care Exercises

Try some of these short exercises while on break to improve your mental, physical, and emotional well-being while at work.

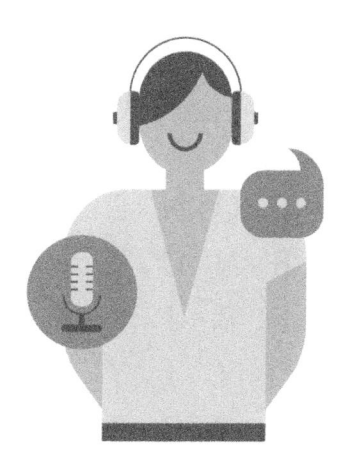

Listen to a podcast to learn new things and viewpoints

Practice a new language to improve brain function and memory

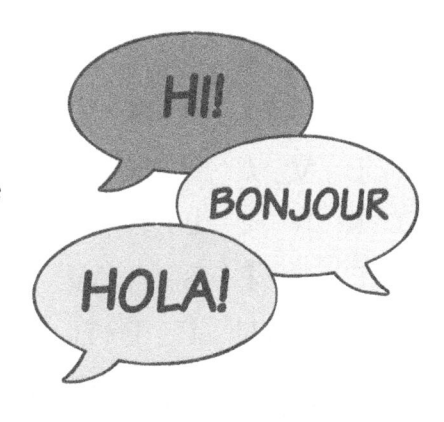

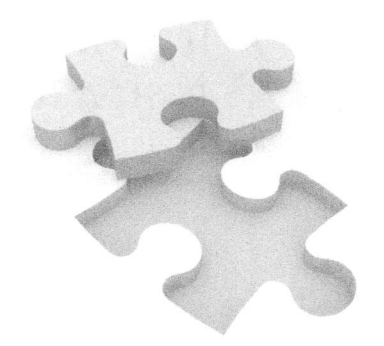

Put a puzzle together to keep your brain sharp and smart

Items Found in a Patient's Room

```
G X F D J L W D F S W E C T H G I L L A C
O S H O J Q V N B Q S C U W P J W M D A I W
R O C V L E N O I T C U S U C M I D E D N N
T E K N A L B N G T N O O T H H T B Q Y I E
L Q A V N G K J B O M K X D R N S A D E C H
X N W D K K G E I E Y O Y Y E S R S N T J M
V D V K R F B S J V S V F I G Q O I C A H R
H R L D K A I E Q Q X I T V V E Q N E G C E
T K Q X C V O Y I T Y A D Q X B N O K M G K
O D W V E B L B B N P B B E B E B J K A Q L
L K A L C O E B E A N B E T T Q Y J Y Y W A
C F E Q N I R V L T T R X D U A U O B I N W
H T M D Y H N F P C I H K T J U B A H J G Q
S A B V A C H A I R H H R M R I G L A D V Y
A D K N L L E W C S P E W O N Y O J E Q Y Y
W A C U E B A W I Q T G K R O S L X B U S F
T D M R N T T H S I H L X I O M H W T R X M
G Q E R D T O O P G Q G W R T O C E J C I G
P D X T A E R M N N I A T R U C D V E B J I
P B O O P T U L E F Y L S P R A H S N T U F
F G J J B C R F K R N G E J N T P H A B S C
Y J U A V E T H E R M O M E T E R U Q G N B
```

BESIDE TABLE	CALL LIGHT	REMOTE	BED
SHEETS	BLANKET	TELEVISION	BATHROOM
DOOR	CHAIR	PATIENT	SUCTION
OXYGEN	THERMOMETER	CURTAIN	WALKER
BASIN	WASHCLOTH	SHARPS	WHITEBOARD

Teamwork!

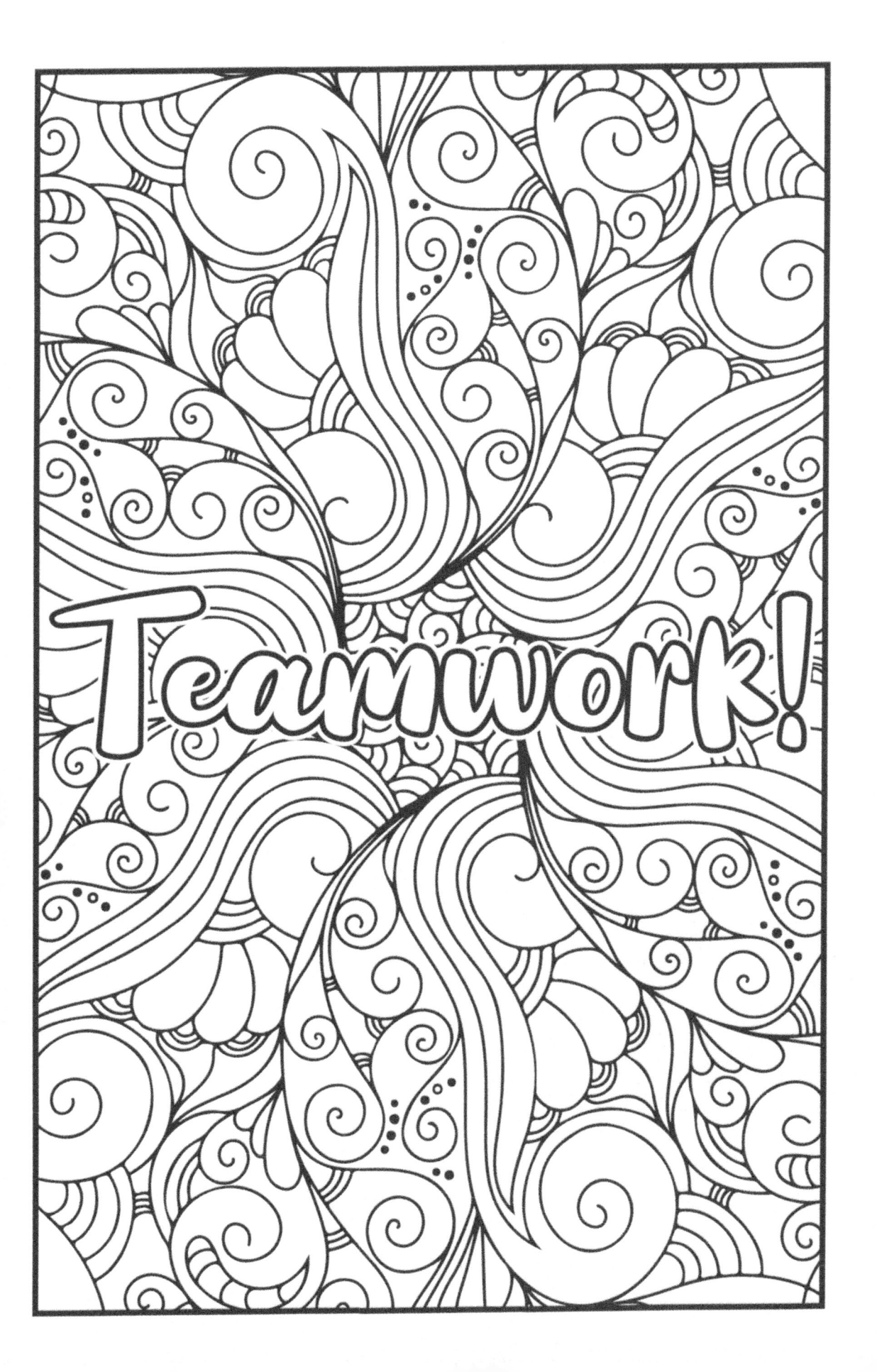

Think about a time when you made a positive impact on a patient's life.

How can you celebrate and honor these moments to remind yourself of the difference you make?

_____
_____
_____
_____
_____
_____
_____
_____
_____
_____
_____
_____
_____
_____
_____
_____
_____
_____

Describe a moment when you felt a deep connection with a patient.

_____
_____
_____
_____
_____
_____
_____
_____
_____
_____
_____
_____
_____
_____
_____
_____
_____
_____
_____

How did that encounter impact you and your sense of purpose in healthcare?

Discuss a patient's journey that profoundly touched your heart.

What lessons did you learn from their experience, and how can you integrate those lessons into your daily practice?

_____
_____
_____
_____
_____
_____
_____
_____
_____
_____
_____
_____
_____
_____
_____
_____
_____
_____

Consider a patient who faced a difficult prognosis. How did you support them emotionally, and how can you apply that same compassion to yourself during challenging times?

Reflect on a mistake you've made in your role. What did you learn from this experience, and how can you transform it into an opportunity for growth and improvement?

Describe a patient interaction that left you feeling emotionally drained.

How can you process your emotions effectively and ensure you're replenishing your emotional reserves?

How can you treat yourself with the kindness and understanding you extend to your patients?

___

TREAT *yourself*

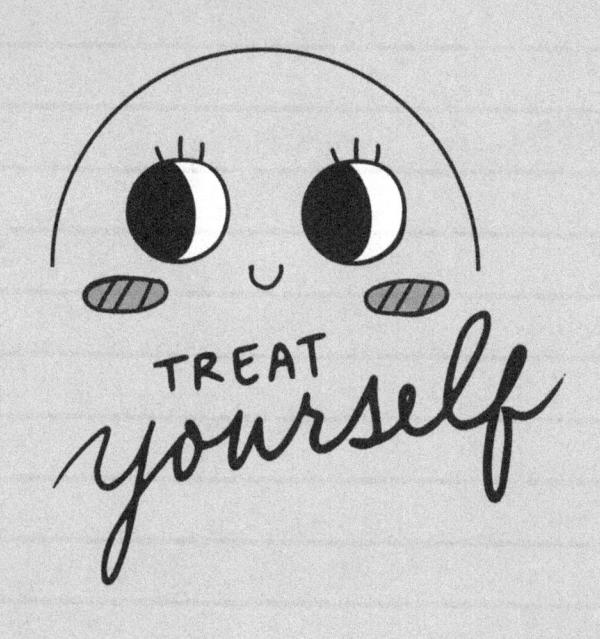

Healthcare Workers

```
D L Y B U B Q N W B D D T C E M O O B D P E
S E M W W M K P H A R M A C I S T K L C E A
F N E A A N U R S E A S S I S T A N T G S A
G U N A I C I N H C E T H T L A E H K M F D
E S R U N D E R E T S I G E R J S B H D R Y
G R K T S I P A R E H T H C E E P S L N C W
G E N U R S E P R A C T I T I O N E R A E H
L N O E G R U S J O S B L D C J G J R W K D
R U T C K U M O U X C N A I C I T E I D P Y
R E T E R P R E T N I L A C I D E M W F W C
P H Y S I C A L T H E R A P I S T C Y F E B
N I D A B F T P S I B N D O C T O R T H R Y
E W Y P A R E H T L A N O I T A P U C C O S
L G W T Q F A U M I D W I F E W K W G R Y J
R A Y E T N A T S I S S A N A I C I S Y H P
E P H A R M A C Y T E C H N I C I A N Q W J
F R B F D B K G S O C I A L W O R K E R W W
L P J N A I C I N H C E T L A C I D E M U G
X V X P R A T I C A L N U R S E F V O B A E
A K N V U G G M L X M H P K F X J L Q T K Y
C K T F D V P V B Y T S I G O L O H C Y S P
T S I P A R E H T Y R O T A R I P S E R T N
```

SOCIAL WORKER	PHYSICAL THERAPIST	REGISTERED NURSE	HEALTH TECHNICIAN
OCCUPATIONAL THERAPY	PHYSICIAN ASSISTANT	RESPIRATORY THERAPIST	PRATICAL NURSE
SPEECH THERAPIST	MEDICAL INTERPRETER	PSYCHOLOGIST	NURSE ASSISTANT
NURSE PRACTITIONER	DOCTOR	MEDICAL TECHNICIAN	PHARMACIST
PHARMACY TECHNICIAN	DIETICIAN	SURGEON	MIDWIFE

"Rehabilitation is the art of reweaving the fabric of a person's life, thread by thread, in a way that supports and empowers them."

-Unknown

DIFFERENCE MAKERS!

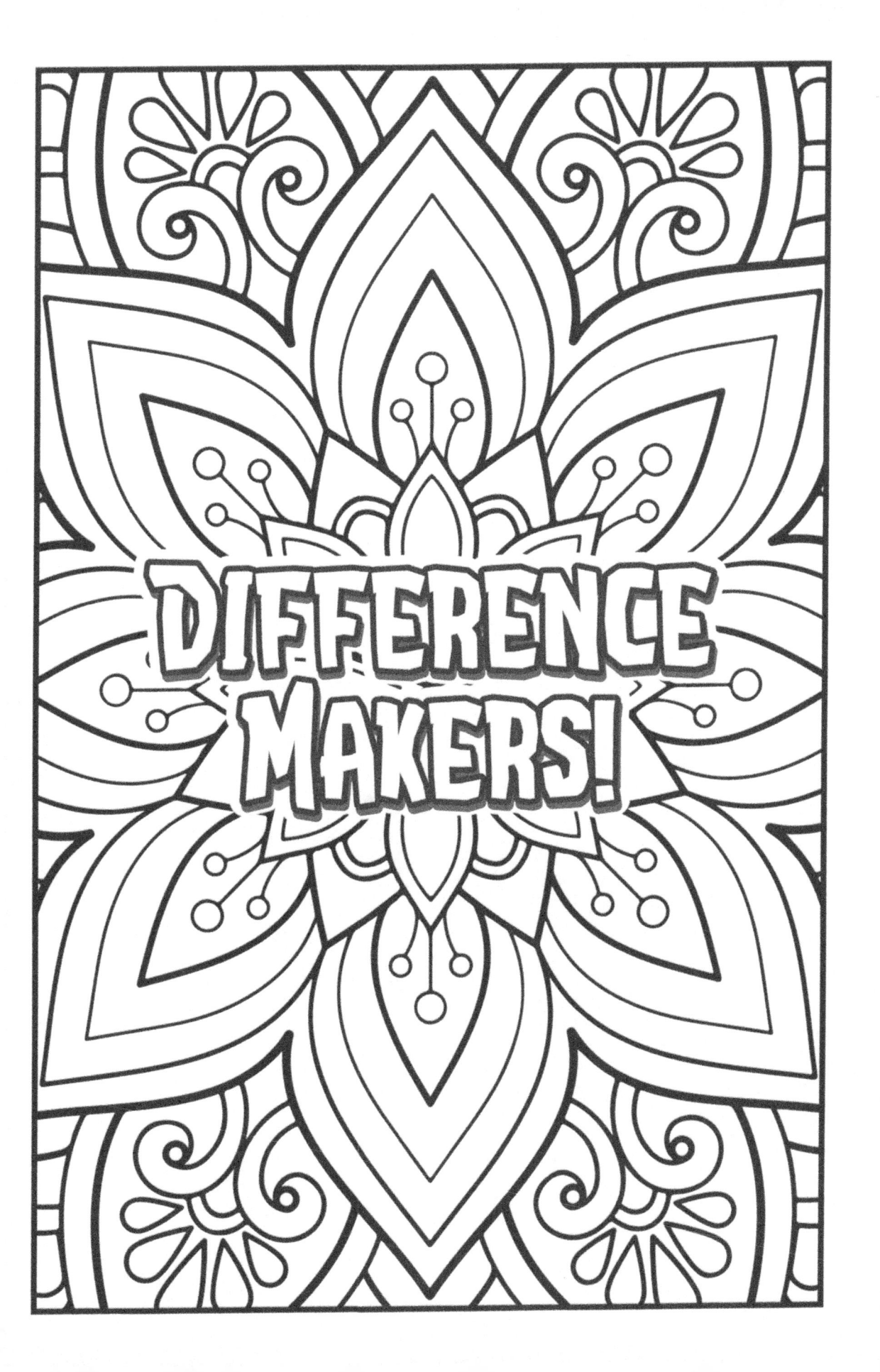

Describe the stigma surrounding mental health in the healthcare field.

How can you contribute to fostering a culture of openness and support within your workplace?

Write about a patient interaction that challenged your beliefs. How did it broaden your interaction?

Describe a moment when you felt proud of a medical decision you made.

___

Reflect on a patient who defied the odds and make a remarkable recovery. How can their story inspire you to persevere through challenges and setbacks?

Describe a time when you felt a disconnect between your personal values and a professional decision. How do you maintain integrity in your role?

What does it mean to you to be a trusted advocate for your patients? How do you maintain that level of trust?

How do you define success as a healthcare professional? It is the lives you save, comfort you provide, or something else?

Image a world where every healthcare professional shares your level of dedication and compassion. What steps can you take to inspire and lead by example?

How do you envision your legacy as a healthcare professional? What mark do you hope to leave on the lives you touched and the field you serve?

If you had to do it all over again, would you still pursue a healthcare career? Why or Why not?

self care

SELF-CARE BINGO

Complete one activity daily, weekly, or monthly

Take a walk during lunch	Dance to your favorite song	Make a new recipe	Listen to a podcast	Treat yourself to a massage
Spend 30 min on a hobby	Read a book	Take a power nap	Sit on porch or under a tree	Eat lunch with a friend
Take a day off social media	Say "NO"	Free Space	Soak in bathtub	Buy yourself something nice
Take the stairs at work	Declutter work bag	Treat yourself to a pedicure	Pack a healthy lunch	Meditation
Go to the salon or barber	Go see a movie	Flirt with your self in the mirror	Color or put together a puzzle	Organize closet or drawer

"The best way to find yourself is to lose yourself in the service of others."

-Mahatma Gandhi

We are one!

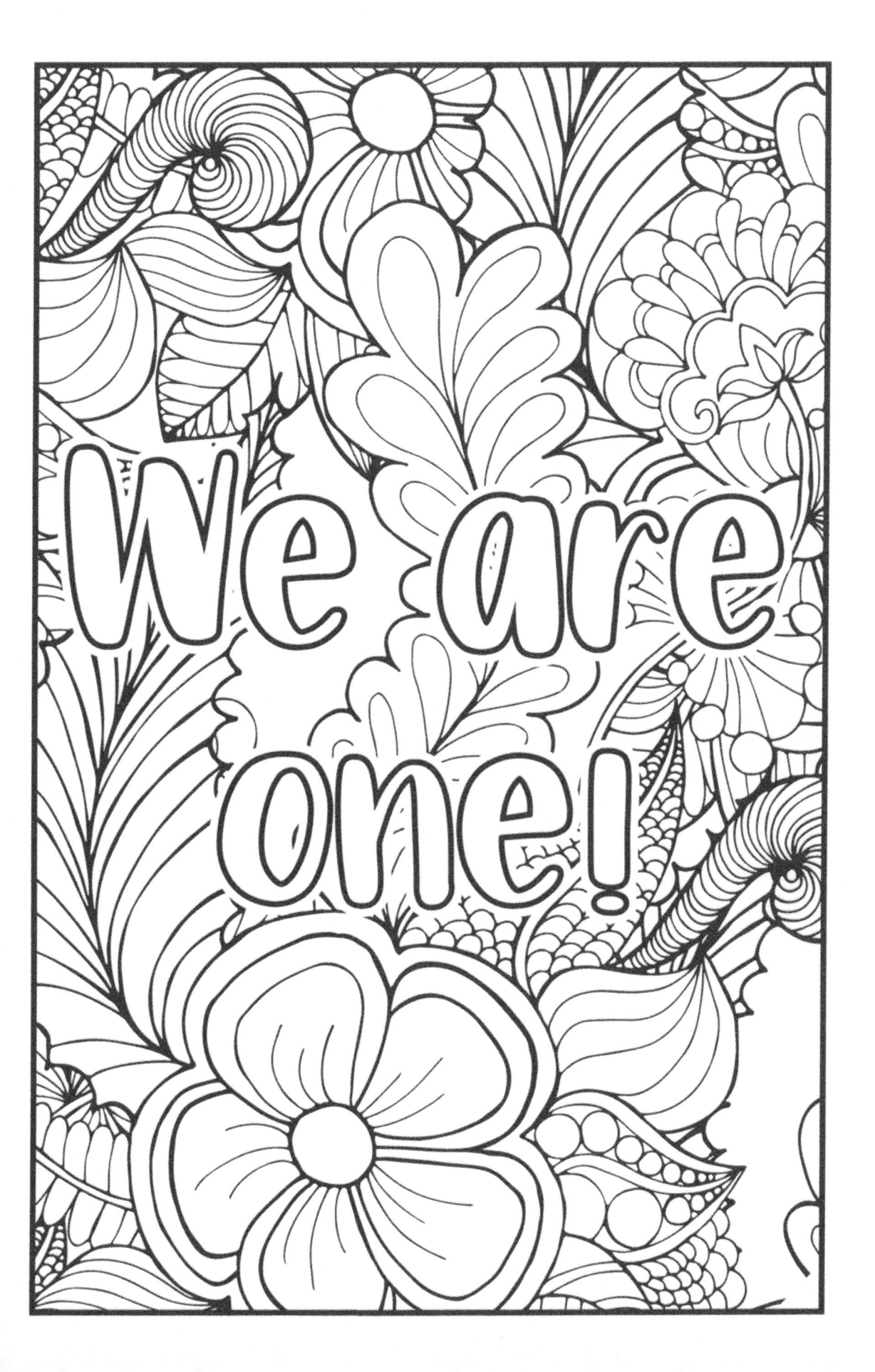

I love my patients!

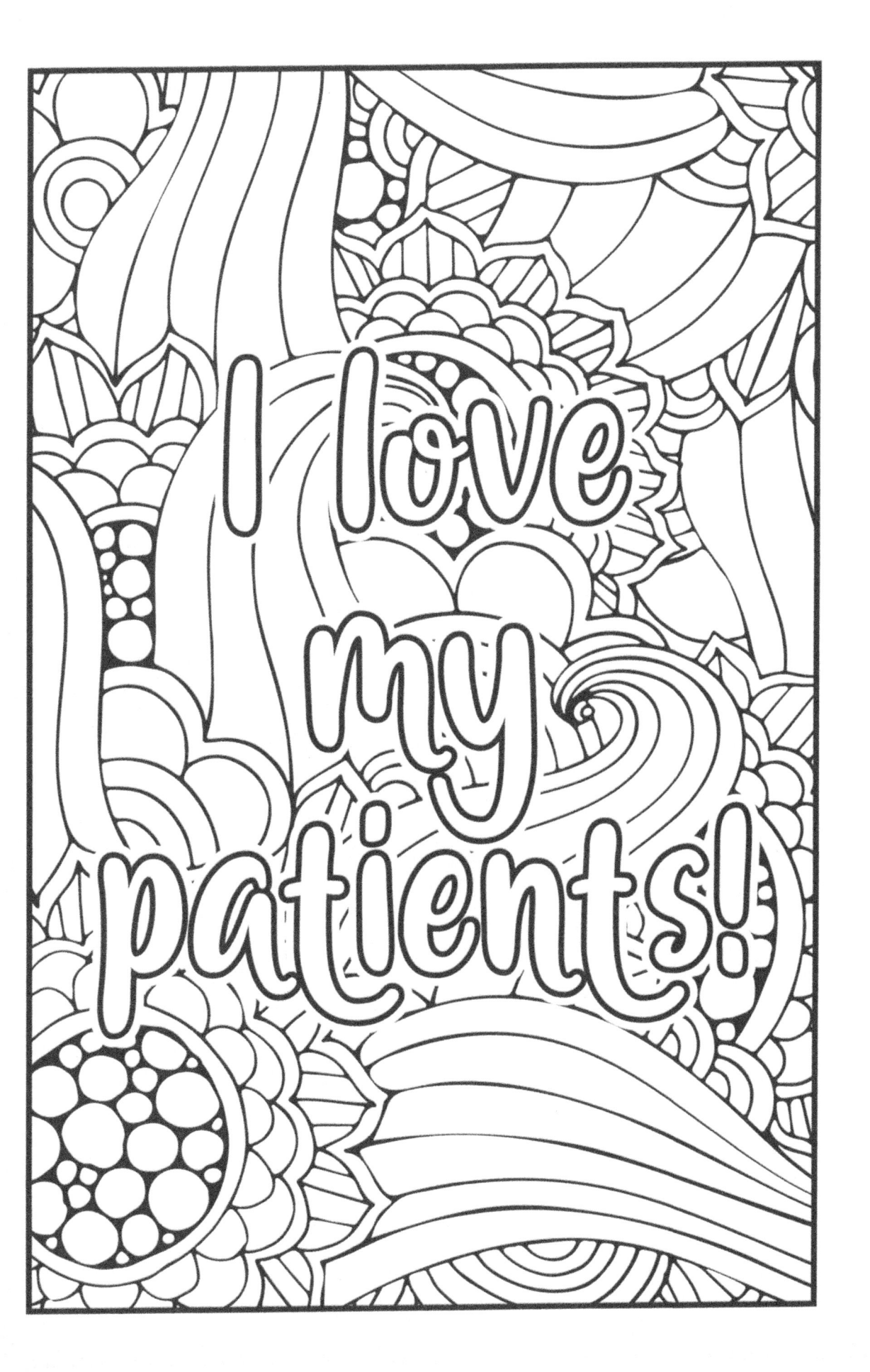

Support Caregivers!

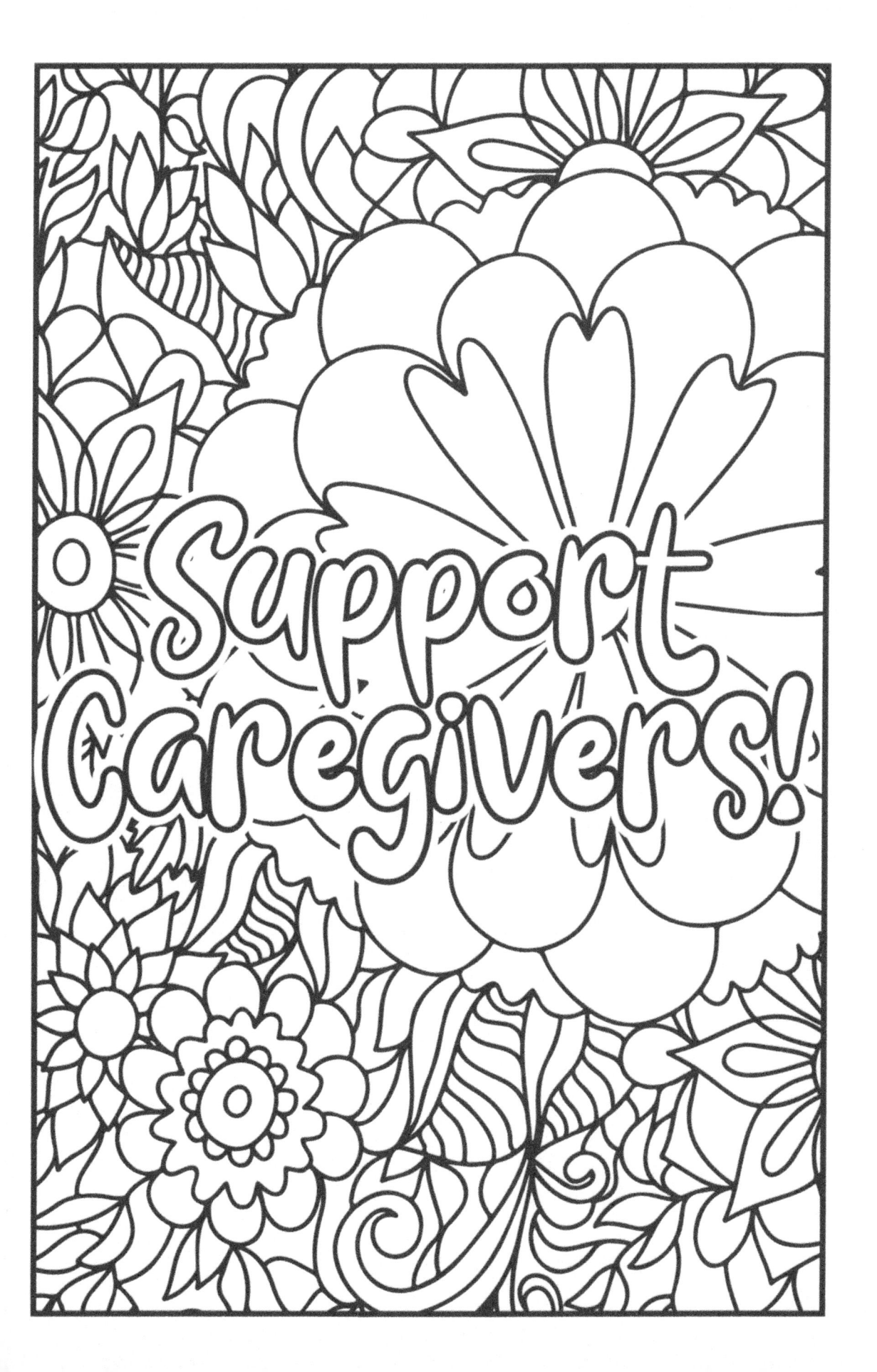

Thank you!

Thank you, the dedicated healthcare professionals who embarked on this journaling adventure. Your commitment to caring for others and nurturing yourselves is genuinely inspiring. I hope the stories, reflections, and moments you've shared within these pages have added new layers of meaning to your profession.

As you continue to navigate the intricate path of healing, may the lessons you've learned within these pages serve as steady guideposts, ensuring that you remain grounded, compassionate, and resilient in the face of all you encounter.

With heartfelt appreciation,

Dr. Tishon Creswell

About the Author

Dr. Tishon Creswell, an award-winning author, seasoned Registered Nurse with 18+ years of experience, a wife, mother, and a proud Army Veteran, currently calls Grovetown, GA, home. Her journey through healthcare is highlighted by her unique blend of compassion and resilience. She has created a transformative journal for fellow healthcare professionals, inviting them to reflect, rekindle their passion, and engage in self-care activities.

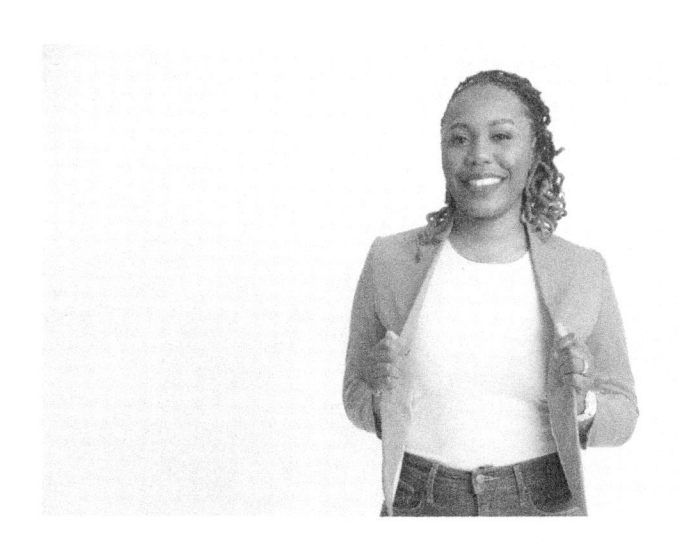

For inquiries and bookings, contact the author at iamtishon@gmail.com
Visit www.iamtishon.com

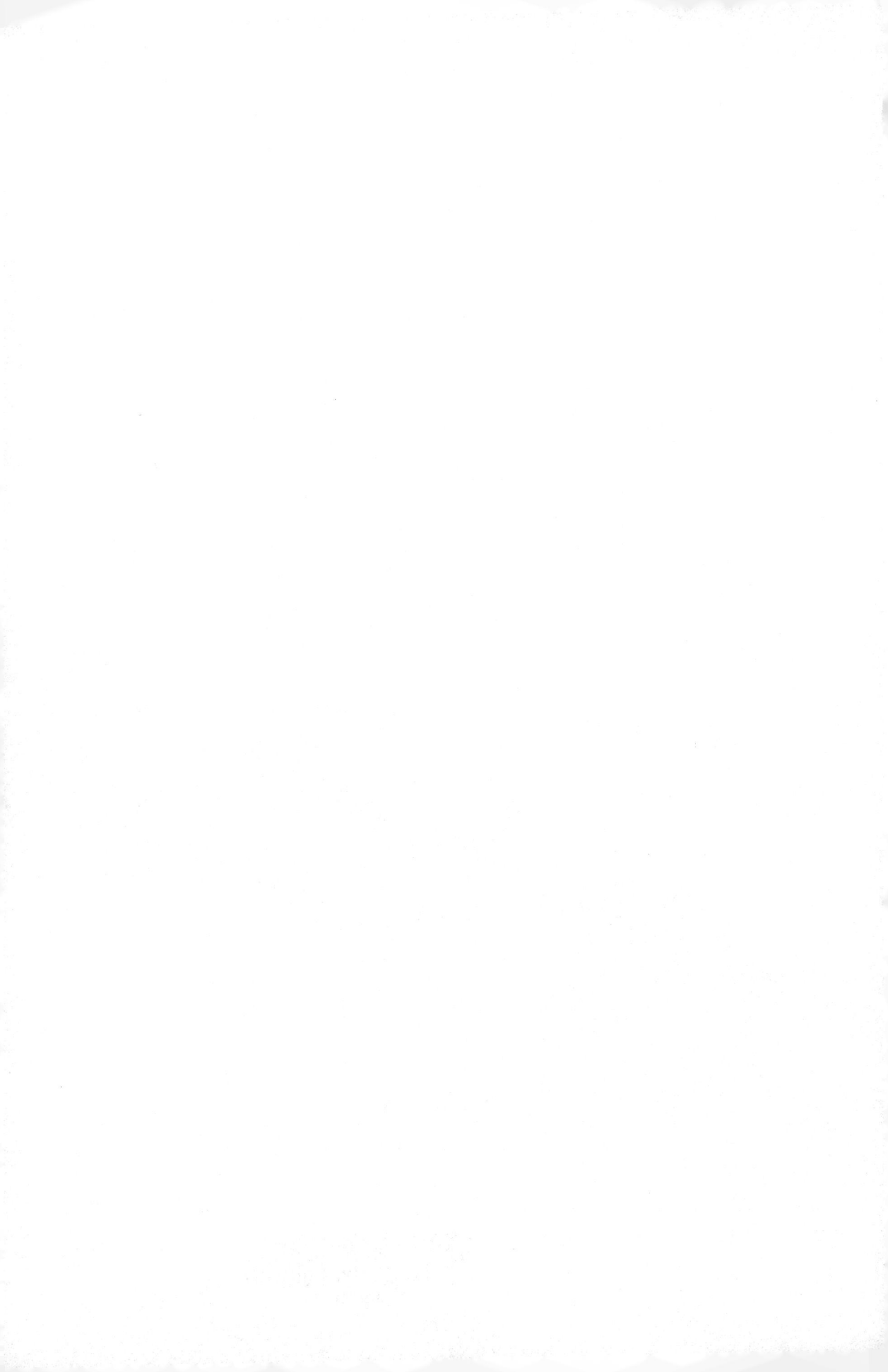

Made in United States
Orlando, FL
22 January 2024